OSTEOPOROSIS DISEASE DIET COOKBOOK

A Comprehensive Guide To Osteoporosis Management Through Nutrition - Recipes, Meal Plans, And Lifestyle Strategies For Optimal Bone Health

Dr. Holmgren Alfred

The content in this book, Osteoporosis Diet Cookbook: is intended solely for educational and informative reasons. This book is not intended to provide medical advice, diagnosis, or treatment. Readers should contact trained healthcare specialists for personalized advice on their specific health conditions and dietary requirements.

The author of this book makes no endorsement, affiliation, or sponsorship of any person, product, website, organization, or other entity mentioned or referenced in the text. Any names, trademarks, or references included in this book are solely for informational purposes and do not constitute endorsement.

Readers are asked to use their discretion and judgment when implementing the nutritional guidelines, recipes, or suggestions contained in this book.

The author and publisher accept no responsibility for any negative effects or repercussions arising from the use or implementation of the material contained herein.

Furthermore, the nutritional guidelines and recipes included in this book may not be appropriate for everyone. Individuals with specific dietary restrictions, allergies, or medical issues should see a healthcare practitioner before making any dietary changes or following the recommendations in this book.

The author and publisher make no warranties or representations about the correctness, completeness, or reliability of the material contained in this book. While every attempt has been made to ensure the material is correct, errors and omissions may occur. The author and publisher are not accountable for any damages or losses resulting from the use of this book.

By reading and utilizing the material contained in this book, readers recognize and agree to the conditions of this disclaimer.

In a society where our health is vital, knowing how to care for our bodies is no longer an option, but a must. Enter the "Osteoporosis Diet Cookbook: With Expert Guidance." This is more than just another cookbook; it's a comprehensive handbook written by experts in the field to help you manage osteoporosis via diet.

This book's central theme is a thorough examination of osteoporosis. What is it? What are the causes and risk factors? These questions are answered, offering a solid foundation on which to build your understanding. But knowledge isn't enough. The book goes on to emphasize the importance of nutrition in the management of osteoporosis. It's more than just eating; it's about supporting your bones and increasing their strength and resilience through wise dietary choices.

Looking through the content, you'll discover a treasure trove of recipes and insights geared at nourishing your bones from breakfast to dinner and everything in between. Whether you're making a calcium-rich breakfast bowl or indulging in a bone-building dessert, each dish is carefully designed to not only satisfy your taste buds but also benefit your skeletal health.

However, it is not only about what you eat; it is also about taking a holistic approach to wellness. The book delves into lifestyle guidelines for healthier bones, including workout recommendations and stress management approaches. It also mentions sunshine exposure for vitamin D production, emphasizing the interconnection of our everyday routines and their effects on bone health.

What distinguishes this work is its practicality. It is not about making major changes or following a rigid diet. Instead, it is about providing you with the knowledge and skills you need to make long-term bone health decisions. This cookbook is more than just recipes; it is about empowerment, allowing you to take control of your health journey with confidence and vigor.

INTRODUCTION

Understanding Osteoporosis.

Osteoporosis is a common skeletal illness characterized by low bone mass and microarchitectural degeneration of bone tissue, resulting in bone fragility and an increased risk of fractures. This illness is a major public health concern around the world, especially among the elderly, because osteoporosis fractures can cause morbidity, disability, and death.

The pathophysiology of osteoporosis involves an imbalance in bone remodeling, in which bone resorption outnumbers bone production, resulting in a net loss of bone mass over time. Several factors can contribute to this imbalance, including hormonal shifts, genetic susceptibility, nutritional inadequacies, and lifestyle choices including smoking and physical inactivity.

What Is Osteoporosis?

Osteoporosis is commonly referred to as a "silent disease" since it usually advances without any obvious signs until a fracture occurs. Fractures associated with osteoporosis are common in the hip, spine, and wrist, and they can be severe, especially in the elderly. Osteoporosis is often diagnosed via bone mineral density testing, such as dual-energy X-ray absorptiometry (DXA), which analyses bone density and determines fracture risk. In addition to low bone mass, osteoporosis can be identified by vertebral abnormalities, decreased height, and postural alterations. Understanding the underlying causes of osteoporosis is critical for creating effective preventative and management methods that reduce its impact on people's health and quality of life.

Causes And Risk Factors

Several variables influence the development of osteoporosis, and understanding these causes and risk factors is critical for risk assessment, prevention, and management. One of the key causes of osteoporosis is age-related bone loss, which occurs when bone mass peaks in early adulthood and gradually falls with age. Hormonal alterations, particularly in postmenopausal women, play an important role in osteoporosis development because lower estrogen levels promote bone loss. Other medical diseases, such as hyperthyroidism, hyperparathyroidism, and gastrointestinal issues, can also impair bone health and raise the risk of osteoporosis.

Lifestyle factors such as sedentary behavior, insufficient physical activity, and poor nutrition are modifiable risk factors for bone health. Nutrition is important in maintaining normal bone density and avoiding osteoporosis because certain nutrients are required for bone production and remodeling. Calcium and vitamin D are two important elements in bone metabolism, with calcium constituting a significant portion of bone tissue and vitamin D promoting calcium absorption and usage. Inadequate calcium and vitamin D intake can hurt bone health and raise the risk of osteoporosis.

Importance Of Nutrition In Osteoporosis Management

Nutrition is critical in the treatment of osteoporosis since dietary choices have a direct impact on bone health and fracture risk. A well-balanced diet rich in key nutrients is critical for maintaining optimal bone density and promoting bone remodeling processes. In addition to calcium and vitamin D, other nutrients such as protein, magnesium, phosphorus, and vitamin K are essential for bone health.

Protein is required for collagen synthesis, which provides the structural framework for bone tissue, whereas magnesium and phosphorus are important components of hydroxyapatite crystals, which help in bone mineralization. Vitamin K is essential for bone metabolism because it regulates calcium binding to bone matrix proteins and stimulates osteoblast activity. Furthermore, antioxidants like vitamins C and E protect bone tissue from oxidative damage and inflammation, which can lead to bone loss and fracture risk. Consuming a variety of nutrient-dense foods, such as dairy products, leafy greens, nuts and seeds, seafood, and fortified meals, can help ensure appropriate consumption of key elements for bone health.

Goals Of Osteoporosis Diet Cookbook

The Osteoporosis Diet Cookbook is intended to give individuals practical advice and resources for implementing dietary recommendations that promote optimal bone health and lower the risk of osteoporosis-related fractures. This thorough guide includes a variety of recipes, food plans, and lifestyle advice aimed at improving bone health and preventing bone loss. The cookbook highlights the significance of eating a well-balanced diet high in calcium, vitamin D, protein, magnesium, phosphorus, and vitamin K.

The cookbook also emphasizes the importance of lifestyle variables like regular physical activity, weight-bearing exercises, and quitting smoking in promoting bone health and lowering fracture risk. The Osteoporosis Diet Cookbook seeks to promote bone health throughout the lifespan by providing consumers with practical tools and information. Finally, the cookbook aims to raise awareness of osteoporosis prevention and management measures, as well as to empower people to make proactive efforts toward preserving strong and healthy bones.

CHAPTER 1
BUILDING STRONG BONES

Maintaining good bone health is critical to general well-being and longevity.

The human skeletal system forms the body's structural structure, giving support, protection, and mobility. However, as individuals age, bone density gradually falls, making them more susceptible to illnesses such as osteoporosis, characterized by weakening and brittle bones. To prevent this degeneration and maintain healthy bones throughout life, it is critical to understand the important nutrients and dietary choices that promote bone health.

Key Nutrients For Bone Health

Calcium: Calcium is probably the most well-known nutrient connected with bone health. It is an essential mineral for the development and maintenance of bone tissue.

Approximately 99% of the body's calcium is stored in bones and teeth, where it gives strength and structure.

Adequate calcium consumption is important to maintain bone mineralization, particularly during years of fast growth, such as in childhood and adolescence, and to avoid bone loss later in life. Good food sources of calcium include dairy products such as milk, cheese, and yogurt, as well as leafy green vegetables like kale and broccoli.

Vitamin D: Vitamin D plays a critical function in calcium absorption and usage throughout the body. It aids in the absorption of dietary calcium from the intestines and helps control calcium levels in the bloodstream.

Additionally, vitamin D is important in bone remodeling, the process by which old bone tissue is replaced by new bone.

Exposure to sunshine is a key source of vitamin D production in the skin, however, it can also be received from dietary sources such as fatty fish (e.g., salmon, mackerel), fortified foods (e.g., fortified milk, breakfast cereals), and pills.

Magnesium: While calcium and vitamin D frequently take center stage in conversations about bone health, magnesium is another key element that helps bone strength and density.

Magnesium has a function in bone development by affecting the activity of osteoblasts, cells responsible for generating new bone structures. Additionally, magnesium helps control calcium metabolism and is involved in the conversion of vitamin D into its active form. Dietary sources of magnesium include nuts, seeds, whole grains, and leafy green vegetables.

Vitamin K: Vitamin K is important for the synthesis of specific proteins involved in bone mineralization and remodeling. Specifically, it accelerates the integration of calcium into bone tissue and helps prevent calcium from accumulating in soft tissues, such as arteries and joints.

There are two basic forms of vitamin K: K1 (phylloquinone), found in green leafy vegetables, and K2 (menaquinone), generated by bacteria in the gut and found in fermented meals and animal products. Both forms contribute to bone health, with vitamin K2 being particularly helpful for reducing calcium buildup in arteries.

Incorporating a range of nutrient-rich foods into the diet is vital for maintaining bone health.

While dairy products are generally linked with calcium, various additional food sources supply vital nutrients for bone health. Leafy green vegetables such as spinach, kale, and collard greens are rich in calcium, magnesium, and vitamin K. Additionally, fortified foods such as plant-based milk alternatives, morning cereals, and orange juice can be helpful sources of calcium and vitamin D for persons who may have dietary restrictions or restricted sun exposure. Fatty fish like salmon and sardines are good providers of both vitamin D and omega-3 fatty acids, which have anti-inflammatory characteristics that may improve bone health.

Recommended Daily Intake Guidelines

The recommended daily consumption of important nutrients for bone health varies depending on characteristics such as age, sex, and individual health status.

For calcium, the recommended dietary allowance (RDA) varies from 1,000 to 1,300 mg per day for most adults, with larger levels advised for adolescents, pregnant and lactating women, and postmenopausal women not receiving estrogen therapy. Vitamin D guidelines also vary but generally range from 600 to 800 international units (IU) per day for adults, with greater doses recommended for persons at risk of insufficiency or with specific medical problems. Magnesium recommendations range from 310 to 420 mg per day for adults, with larger levels suggested during pregnancy and lactation. Lastly, vitamin K guidelines are often given as acceptable intake (AI) values, which vary from 90 to 120 mcg per day for people. However, it is necessary to contact a healthcare practitioner to evaluate personalized nutrient needs and to ensure optimal bone health through the right nutrition and lifestyle choices.

CHAPTER 2
BREAKFASTS FOR BONE HEALTH

Breakfast is typically praised as the most important meal of the day, and for individuals trying to maintain or improve bone health, it gives a key opportunity to jumpstart the day with nutrient-dense foods that boost skeletal strength.

This section of the "Osteoporosis Diet Cookbook" dives into the relevance of breakfast in the context of bone health and presents a profusion of breakfast options customized specifically to boost bone density and general skeletal health. Recognizing that breakfast sets the tone for the day's nutritional intake, the recipes and meal ideas presented here prioritize components rich in critical bone-building elements such as calcium, vitamin D, and protein.

By prioritizing the inclusion of these critical nutrients in the morning meal, individuals can establish a solid foundation for good bone health throughout the day.

Nutrient-Rich Breakfast Recipes:

Nutrient-rich breakfast meals constitute the cornerstone of a bone-healthy morning routine. This chapter of the cookbook introduces readers to a broad assortment of breakfast options painstakingly created to give a robust dosage of critical vitamins and minerals important for keeping strong and resilient bones.

From hearty whole-grain porridge topped with calcium-rich almonds and seeds to protein-packed Greek yogurt parfaits decked with vitamin D-rich fruits, these recipes prioritize nutritious, unprocessed ingredients that nourish the body from within.

By including nutrient-rich foods in breakfast meals, consumers may ensure they start their day on a fortified note, setting the stage for ongoing bone health and vigor.

Calcium-Rich Breakfast Bowls:

Calcium, a mineral famous for its role in bone production and preservation, takes center stage in breakfast bowls designed to boost skeletal strength.

This chapter of the cookbook explores a variety of calcium-rich breakfast bowl recipes that effortlessly incorporate dairy and non-dairy sources of this key nutrient. From creamy Greek yogurt bowls topped with fresh fruit and crunchy granola to calcium-fortified smoothie bowls filled with leafy greens and nuts, these breakfast concoctions offer a delightful and simple manner of satisfying daily calcium requirements. By choosing calcium-rich breakfast options, individuals can maximize bone health and reduce the risk of osteoporosis, ensuring that each spoonful adds to the strength and durability of their skeletal foundation.

Vitamin D Boosting Smoothies:

Vitamin D, often lauded as the "sunshine vitamin," plays a vital function in calcium absorption and bone mineralization.

In this section of the cookbook, readers are introduced to vitamin D-boosting smoothie recipes created to harness the nutritional power of this crucial nutrient.

These smoothies, which combine fortified dairy or plant-based milk, leafy greens, and vitamin D-enriched fruits, provide a refreshing and delightful way to support bone health. Whether consumed as a solitary breakfast option or mixed with other bone-nourishing meals, these vitamin D-packed smoothies provide a handy alternative for individuals aiming to improve their skeletal health and resilience.

Fortified Breakfast Cereals:

Breakfast cereals, a beloved morning staple for many, undergo a radical makeover in this part of the cookbook, emerging as fortified powerhouses of bone-supporting minerals. Recognizing the broad popularity and convenience of breakfast cereals, this section showcases a range of fortified cereal options specifically chosen for their capacity to contribute to optimal bone health. Whether whole-grain flakes loaded with calcium and vitamin D or fortified oat clusters teeming with bone-nourishing nuts and seeds, these cereals offer a straightforward and accessible manner of reinforcing the morning meal with key elements required for skeletal strength.

By including fortified breakfast cereals into their morning routine, individuals may effortlessly raise their intake of bone-supporting vitamins and minerals, setting the stage for enhanced skeletal health and resilience.

Omelets With Leafy Greens:

Omelets, with their adaptable character and capacity to accommodate several healthy fillings, emerge as a savory answer for enhancing bone health in this portion of the cookbook. By integrating leafy greens such as spinach, kale, or collard greens into omelette recipes, folks may infuse their morning meal with a robust dose of bone-strengthening elements, including calcium, vitamin K, and magnesium.

Whether consumed as a solitary breakfast choice or combined with whole-grain toast and fresh fruit, these leafy green omelettes offer a tasty and pleasant manner of boosting bone health. With each forkful, people may enjoy the synergy of healthy nutrients working together to promote good bone health and resilience.

Tips For Improving Bone Health With Breakfast Meals:

Aside from a profusion of bone-healthy breakfast recipes, this portion of the cookbook provides readers with practical suggestions and tactics for improving bone health in their morning meals.

From incorporating calcium-rich foods like dairy products, fortified plant-based alternatives, and leafy greens to ensuring adequate vitamin D intake through fortified foods or supplementation, these suggestions provide actionable advice for maximizing breakfast's bone-nourishing potential. Furthermore, pairing calcium-rich foods with sources of vitamin D and vitamin K improves nutrient absorption and bone mineralization, boosting breakfast's effectiveness in maintaining skeletal strength and resilience. Individuals who include these evidence-based methods in their morning routine can embark on a journey to enhanced bone health and a lower risk of osteoporosis, one tasty meal at a time.

CHAPTER 3
NUTRITIONAL LUNCHES

The term "nourishing lunches" encapsulates the pivotal role of midday meals in fostering optimal bone health and overall well-being. A balanced lunch not only satisfies hunger but also provides essential nutrients crucial for bone density maintenance and osteoporosis management. The concept of balanced lunch recipes emphasizes the importance of incorporating a variety of food groups to ensure a comprehensive nutrient intake.

"Calcium-packed salads" represent a sophisticated yet accessible approach to augmenting calcium intake, a cornerstone of osteoporosis management. Salads, typically revered for their refreshing qualities, transform with the incorporation of calcium-rich ingredients, elevating them into potent allies in bone health.

The concept underscores the versatility of salads as a canvas for incorporating diverse calcium sources such as leafy greens, fortified tofu, almonds, and dairy products like cheese or yogurt.

Beyond merely fortifying salads with calcium-rich foods, attention is also directed towards maximizing bioavailability through strategic pairing with vitamin D sources, which facilitate calcium absorption.

This synergy ensures that the body can efficiently utilize the ingested calcium, thereby optimizing its bone-strengthening effects. By reinventing salads as vehicles for delivering essential bone nutrients, individuals can seamlessly integrate them into their dietary repertoire, fostering a sustainable approach to osteoporosis management.

"Grilled Fish Tacos with Avocado" epitomizes the fusion of culinary delight with nutritional prowess, offering a delectable yet nourishing lunch option. Beyond its gastronomic appeal, this concept underscores the importance of incorporating omega-3 fatty acids, protein, and micronutrients like vitamin D and magnesium, all of which contribute to bone health. Fish, particularly varieties like salmon, sardines, and mackerel, serve as an exemplary source of omega-3 fatty acids, renowned for their anti-inflammatory properties and potential to mitigate bone loss. Coupled with avocado, which not only enhances the flavor profile but also supplies monounsaturated fats and potassium, this dish exemplifies a harmonious marriage of taste and nutrition. The inclusion of vitamin D-rich ingredients like grilled mushrooms or fortified tortillas further amplifies its bone-supportive benefits. Through innovative culinary creations such as grilled fish tacos with avocado, individuals can savor a culinary delight while fortifying their skeletal integrity, thereby transcending the conventional dichotomy between indulgence and health.

"Vegetable Quinoa Bowls" epitomize the synergy between plant-based nutrition and bone health, offering a nutrient-dense and versatile lunch option. At the core of this concept lies quinoa, a pseudo-grain celebrated for its complete protein profile and abundance of bone-bolstering nutrients such as magnesium, phosphorus, and manganese. Complemented by an array of colorful vegetables like kale, bell peppers, and carrots, these bowls are replete with antioxidants, vitamins, and minerals crucial for bone metabolism and overall vitality.

The incorporation of legumes or tofu further augments the protein content, while nuts and seeds contribute healthy fats and additional micronutrients. By embracing vegetable quinoa bowls, individuals not only partake in a culinary journey bursting with flavors and textures but also fortify their skeletal framework through the amalgamation of diverse plant-based nutrients. This concept underscores the adaptability of plant-centric diets in fulfilling the multifaceted requirements of osteoporosis management, advocating for a holistic approach to nutrition and bone health.

"Broccoli and Cheese Stuffed Chicken Breasts" epitomize the amalgamation of wholesome ingredients and culinary ingenuity, offering a savory and nutrient-rich lunch option conducive to bone health. Central to this concept is the strategic pairing of lean protein from chicken breasts with calcium-rich broccoli and cheese, creating a symphony of flavors and nutrients.

Broccoli emerges as a nutritional powerhouse, boasting an array of bone-strengthening nutrients such as calcium, vitamin K, and sulforaphane, a compound with potential anti-inflammatory and bone-protective properties.

Coupled with calcium-rich cheese, which provides not only flavor but also essential nutrients like protein and phosphorus, this dish exemplifies a harmonious marriage of taste and nutrition. The incorporation of lean protein from chicken breasts ensures satiety and muscle maintenance, further augmenting its nutritional appeal.

 By embracing innovative culinary creations such as broccoli and cheese stuffed chicken breasts, individuals can savor a wholesome meal while fortifying their skeletal integrity, thereby transcending the conventional notion of restrictive diets in osteoporosis management.

CHAPTER 4
DINNER DELIGHTS

This section of the "Osteoporosis Diet Cookbook" emphasizes the importance of wholesome dinner options that are not only delicious but also rich in

Wholesome Dinner Options:

The "Osteoporosis Diet Cookbook" is a collection of nutritious dinner recipes that cater to a variety of tastes and preferences. From the succulent Baked Salmon with Lemon and Herbs to the vibrant Tofu Stir-Fry with Vegetables, each recipe offers a distinct combination of ingredients that contribute to

Cooking Techniques for Preserving Bone-Beneficial Nutrients

While the selection of bone-healthy ingredients is pivotal in dinner preparation, the choice of cooking techniques plays an equally significant role in preserving the nutritional value of these ingredients.

The "Osteoporosis Diet Cookbook" underscores the importance of adopting cooking methods that retain bone-beneficial nutrients while enhancing the flavor and texture of the dishes. Techniques such as baking, steaming, and stir-frying are emphasized for their ability to minimize nutrient loss during the cooking process. For instance, baking salmon with lemon and herbs preserves its omega-3 fatty acids, which are essential for bone health, while steaming vegetables in a tofu stir-fry ensures that water-soluble vitamins like vitamin C are retained. Additionally, the use of minimal oil and salt in cooking helps to promote heart health and mitigate the risk of conditions that could exacerbate bone loss, aligning with comprehensive osteoporosis management through nutrition. By adopting these cooking techniques, individuals can maximize the nutritional benefits of their dinner meals, thereby supporting their journey toward optimal bone health.

These paragraphs provide in-depth insights into the concepts of Dinner Delights, Wholesome Dinner Options, and Cooking Techniques to Preserve Bone-Beneficial Nutrients, as outlined in the "Osteoporosis Diet Cookbook." Each concept is discussed in an academic tone, emphasizing the importance of incorporating nutrient-rich ingredients and using appropriate cooking methods in the pursuit of optimal bone health.

CHAPTER 5
SNACKS AND SMALL BITES

Snacks and small bites play a significant role in providing essential nutrients that contribute to bone strength and integrity. These intermediate meals, often consumed between larger meals, offer opportunities to incorporate various food groups crucial for bone health, such as calcium, vitamin D, protein, and other essential micronutrients. Despite their smaller portion size, snacks can be strategically designed.

Nutritional Snack Ideas:

Among the plethora of snack options available, some stand out for their ability to deliver a combination of nutrients beneficial for bone health. Greek yogurt with nuts and berries presents a potent blend of calcium from yogurt, protein from nuts, and antioxidants from berries, offering a wholesome snack that supports bone strength and overall health. Similarly, cheese and whole grain crackers offer a convenient way to incorporate calcium-rich dairy along with

The Importance Of Snacking For Bone Health:

The significance of snacking in the context of bone health stems from its role in sustaining a steady supply of essential nutrients throughout the day. Unlike main meals, which may be spaced several hours apart, snacks bridge the nutritional gap between meals, preventing prolonged periods of nutrient deprivation that can negatively impact bone metabolism.

By incorporating nutrient-rich snacks into one's daily eating pattern, individuals can ensure a consistent intake of calcium, vitamin D, protein, and other micronutrients crucial for bone formation, repair, and maintenance. Moreover, snacking can help regulate blood sugar levels and prevent overeating during main meals, promoting overall dietary balance and metabolic health, factors that indirectly contribute to bone health. For individuals with osteoporosis or those at risk of developing the condition, strategic snacking can serve as a practical tool for optimizing nutrient intake and supporting bone health goals, complementing other lifestyle interventions such as exercise and medication adherence.

 The osteoporosis diet cookbook takes a holistic approach to managing bone health through nutrition, emphasizing the importance of snacking for bone health and offering a variety of nutritious snack ideas. The cookbook's goal is to provide individuals with practical strategies for incorporating bone-supportive nutrients into their daily eating habits.

CHAPTER 6
BONE-BUILDING DESSERTS

Bone health is a critical aspect of overall well-being, with conditions such as osteoporosis necessitating diligent attention and proactive measures. While dietary interventions are often associated with savory dishes and nutrient-dense meals, the concept of bone-building desserts introduces a novel approach to integrating essential nutrients into one's diet. Desserts, which are typically perceived as indulgent and potentially detrimental to health, can be transformed into

Healthy Dessert Recipes:

In a society where desserts are commonly associated with excess sugar, unhealthy fats, and empty calories, the emergence of recipes tailored to promote well-being marks a paradigm shift in culinary culture.

Berry Parfaits With Greek Yogurt

Berries like strawberries, blueberries, and raspberries are renowned for their antioxidant properties and high content of vitamins C and K, minerals like manganese, and phytonutrients like anthocyanins. Greek yogurt, prized for its richness in calcium

Dark Chocolate-Dipped Fruit

Dark chocolate, with its high cocoa content, is a rich source of flavonoids, particularly flavanols, which have been linked to improved cardiovascular health and increased bone density. When paired with fruits like strawberries, bananas, or oranges, dark chocolate not only adds depth to the flavor profile but also contributes.

Chia Seed Pudding With Almond Milk

Chia seed pudding with almond milk is a versatile dessert option that marries convenience with nutritional excellence. Chia seeds, revered for their omega-3 fatty acid content, fiber, and calcium, form the foundation of this dessert, providing a nutrient-dense base that promotes bone health. Almond milk, a dairy alternative enriched with vitamin E and calcium, lends creaminess to the pudding while further enhancing its nutritional profile. Chia seeds absorb

Baked Apples With Cinnamon And Walnuts.

Baked apples with cinnamon and walnuts exemplify the marriage of simplicity and sophistication in dessert preparation.

This classic dessert combines the natural sweetness of apples with the warm, aromatic notes of cinnamon and the earthy crunch of walnuts, resulting in a harmonious medley of flavors and textures.

Indulge Smartly: Sweets For Bone Health

Indulging wisely entails navigating the realm of sweets with mindfulness and intentionality, recognizing that indulgence can coexist with health-conscious choices. Sweets for bone health encompass a spectrum of desserts crafted with a keen awareness of nutritional principles and their implications for skeletal integrity.

CHAPTER 7
BEVERAGES FOR BONE STRENGTH

Adequate hydration is essential for optimal bone function because water makes up a significant portion of bone composition. Dehydration can lead to a decrease in bone density and mineralization, making bones more susceptible to fractures and osteoporosis, so maintaining proper hydration levels is paramount for bone strength and integrity.

Bone-Boosting Drink Recipes:

Green smoothies with kale and pineapple are a popular beverage choice for individuals looking to boost their intake of vitamins, minerals, and antioxidants, all of which are crucial for bone health. Kale, a leafy green vegetable rich in calcium, vitamin K, and other bone-strengthening nutrients, serves as a key ingredient in green smoothies. Pineapple adds a touch of sweetness and provides additional nutrients, such as vitamin C, which plays a vital role.

Calcium-fortified plant-based milk, such as almond milk, soy milk, and oat milk, are excellent sources of calcium, vitamin D, and other nutrients essential for bone health. These dairy-free alternatives are especially beneficial for individuals who are lactose intolerant or follow a vegan lifestyle.

Herbal teas have long been praised for their medicinal properties and health benefits, including support for bone health. Certain herbs, such as nettle leaf, horsetail, red clover, and alfalfa, contain compounds that promote bone formation, inhibit bone breakdown, and reduce inflammation, all of which contribute to the maintenance of strong and healthy bones.

 Calcium-Rich Fruit Juices: Fruit juices can be a convenient and tasty way to increase calcium intake and support bone health, especially for individuals who may struggle to consume dairy products or other calcium-rich foods. Certain fruits, such as oranges, figs, and fortified juices, contain significant amounts of calcium, along with vitamins and minerals that contribute to bone health. Oranges, for example, are not only high in vitamin C but also contain calcium and magnesium.

CHAPTER 8
MEAL PLANNING AND STRATEGIES

Individuals diagnosed with osteoporosis must adopt dietary strategies that promote optimal bone health, ensuring an adequate intake of essential nutrients crucial for bone density and strength. To support bone health while also addressing overall nutritional needs, effective meal planning involves meticulous consideration of nutrient composition, portion sizes, and meal frequency.

Tips for Planning Meals with Osteoporosis:

1. For individuals with osteoporosis, calcium and vitamin D-rich foods are essential for bone mineralization and calcium homeostasis. Dairy products like milk, yogurt, and cheese are high in

calcium, while fatty fish like salmon and sardines are high in vitamin D. Fortified foods, such as orange juice and cereals, can also help meet daily requirements.

2. Incorporate Plant-Based Sources: Plant-based foods like tofu, kale, broccoli, and fortified plant-based milk can provide significant amounts of calcium. Additionally, a diverse nutrient profile, including magnesium, potassium, and vitamin K, is important for bone health.

To maintain bone density, individuals with osteoporosis should limit their intake of processed foods high in sodium and limit their consumption of caffeinated beverages like coffee and tea. Instead, opt for healthier alternatives such as herbal teas or decaffeinated options.

To maintain muscle mass and bone health, individuals should aim for moderate protein intake, including lean protein sources such as poultry, fish, legumes, and nuts. Excessive protein intake, especially from animal sources, may increase calcium excretion.

Magnesium and vitamin K are essential cofactors in bone metabolism and play crucial roles in bone mineralization. Magnesium is found in green leafy vegetables, nuts, seeds, and whole grains, while vitamin K is abundant in leafy greens like spinach, kale, and Brussels sprouts. Incorporating these foods into meal plans can optimize bone health.

Creating Balanced Meals:

1. To support bone health, include high-calcium foods in each meal, such as dairy products like milk or yogurt, calcium-fortified foods like tofu or cereals, or non-

dairy options like leafy greens, almonds, and sesame seeds.

2. Include Lean Protein Sources: Lean protein sources including poultry, fish, beans, lentils, and tofu can help maintain muscle and bone health while reducing saturated fat intake.

Whole grains, such as brown rice, quinoa, oats, and whole-grain bread, are rich in nutrients such as magnesium and B vitamins, which are beneficial for bone health. Their high fiber content also aids digestion and nutrient absorption.

4. Consume a Variety of Colorful Fruits and Vegetables: Fruits and vegetables contain essential vitamins, minerals, and antioxidants for overall health. Dark leafy greens like spinach and kale are especially beneficial for bone mineralization due to their high vitamin K content.

5. Consume healthy unsaturated fats in moderation, such as olive oil, avocado, nuts, and seeds, to offer vital fatty acids without affecting bone health.

Sample Weekly Meal Plans:

A well-structured meal plan can help individuals adhere to dietary recommendations for managing osteoporosis while enjoying a diverse range of foods. Sample meal plans provide practical guidance for individuals with osteoporosis to structure their daily dietary intake effectively and ensure adequate nutrient intake while promoting variety and flexibility in food choices.

Day 1:

- Breakfast: Greek yogurt with sliced almonds and mixed berries, served with whole-grain toast.

- Lunch: Spinach and kale salad with grilled chicken, quinoa, cherry tomatoes, and balsamic vinaigrette dressing.

- Snack: Carrot sticks with hummus.

- Dinner: Baked salmon, steamed broccoli, brown rice.

Day 2:

- Breakfast: Spinach and feta omelette with whole-grain English muffins.

- Lunch: Lentil soup, mixed green salad, and whole grain bun.

- Snack: Apple slices and almond butter.

- Dinner: Stir-fried tofu with bell peppers and snap peas, served over brown rice.

Day 3:

- Breakfast: Overnight oatmeal with rolled oats, chia seeds, almond milk, sliced bananas, and walnuts.

• Lunch option: Turkey and avocado wrap with lettuce, tomato, and whole grain tortilla.

• Snack: Greek yogurt, honey, and sliced peaches.

• Dinner: Quinoa stuffed bell peppers with black beans, corn, tomatoes, and avocado.

Day 4:

• Breakfast: Whole grain waffles with Greek yogurt and mixed berries.

• Lunch: Grilled shrimp Caesar salad with romaine, cherry tomatoes, Parmesan cheese, and whole-grain croutons.

• Snack: Cottage cheese with pineapple chunks

• Dinner: Baked chicken breast with roasted sweet potatoes and steamed green beans

Day 5:

• Breakfast: Smoothie made with spinach, banana, almond milk, and protein powder

• Lunch: Chickpea salad with cucumber, tomatoes, feta cheese, olives, and lemon-tahini dressing

• Snack: Trail mix with mixed nuts and dry fruit

• Dinner: Beef stir-fry with broccoli, bell peppers, and snow peas served over brown rice

Day 6:

• Breakfast: Whole-grain pancakes topped with Greek yogurt and sliced strawberries

• Lunch: Quinoa salad with roasted veggies (zucchini, bell peppers, eggplant) and feta cheese

• Snack: Edamame pods

- Dinner: Baked cod with asparagus and wild rice pilaf

Day 7:

- Breakfast: Scrambled eggs with sautéed spinach and whole-grain bread

- Lunch: Caprese salad with fresh mozzarella, tomatoes, basil, drizzled with balsamic sauce, and whole-grain baguette

- Snack: Cottage cheese with sliced pear

- Dinner: Vegetable and tofu curry with brown rice

These sample meal plans provide a blueprint for individuals with osteoporosis to structure their meals throughout the week, ensuring adequate intake of essential nutrients while promoting variety and enjoyment in eating. It's essential to personalize meal plans based on individual dietary preferences, cultural considerations, and specific health needs while adhering to general guidelines for osteoporosis management through nutrition. Regular consultation with a registered dietitian or healthcare professional can further optimize meal planning strategies tailored to individual requirements and goals.

CHAPTER 9
SHOPPING AND STOCKING YOUR KITCHEN

When embarking on the journey of managing osteoporosis through nutrition, one of the fundamental steps is to optimize your kitchen space to support bone health. This entails strategic shopping and stocking practices to ensure that your pantry and refrigerator are brimming with essential ingredients conducive to bone strength and overall well-being.

Shopping for a bone-healthy kitchen involves a multifaceted approach, encompassing ingredient selection, nutritional awareness, and mindful consumption. It's not merely about filling your shelves with food items but rather about curating a collection of nutrient-rich foods tailored to support bone health.

Essential Ingredients for a Bone-Healthy Kitchen:

Central to the concept of a bone-healthy kitchen are the essential ingredients that serve as the building blocks for nutritious meals aimed at fortifying bones and combating osteoporosis.

These ingredients typically comprise a diverse array of foods rich in calcium, vitamin D, vitamin K, magnesium, and other micronutrients crucial for bone metabolism and strength.

Calcium-rich foods such as dairy products, leafy greens, fortified plant-based milk, and canned fish with bones are pivotal in promoting bone density and resilience. Vitamin D sources, including fatty fish, egg yolks, and fortified foods, facilitate calcium absorption and play a vital role in bone health.

Additionally, vitamin K from leafy greens, cruciferous vegetables, and fermented foods contributes to bone mineralization and reduces fracture risk. Magnesium, found abundantly in nuts, seeds, whole grains, and legumes, supports bone structure and function by aiding in calcium absorption and retention. Incorporating these essential ingredients into daily culinary endeavors lays a solid foundation for fostering optimal bone health and mitigating the effects of osteoporosis.

Smart Shopping Tips:

Navigating the aisles of grocery stores with a discerning eye is paramount when striving to assemble a bone-healthy kitchen. Smart shopping entails strategic decision-making regarding ingredient selection, label reading, and budget-conscious choices. Prioritizing fresh, whole foods over processed alternatives ensures a higher intake of vital nutrients essential for bone health. Focusing on nutrient-dense items such as fruits, vegetables, lean proteins, and whole grains not only fortifies bones but also promotes overall wellness.

When selecting packaged foods, scrutinizing nutrition labels for calcium, vitamin D, and other bone-supporting nutrients aids in making informed choices.

Opting for products fortified with these essential nutrients can supplement dietary intake and enhance bone health. Additionally, leveraging seasonal produce and sales promotions can optimize cost-effectiveness without compromising nutritional quality. By adhering to these smart shopping tips, individuals can effectively stock their kitchens with bone-nourishing foods while making prudent financial decisions.

Building a robust repertoire of bone-building foods is a cornerstone of effective osteoporosis management through nutrition. Stocking up on a variety of nutrient-rich foods ensures culinary versatility and dietary adequacy, thereby empowering individuals to craft balanced meals tailored to their bone health needs. Staples such as dairy products, leafy greens, nuts, seeds, whole grains, and lean proteins should feature prominently in the kitchen inventory. Fresh produce should be prioritized whenever feasible, but frozen and canned options can also serve as convenient alternatives without compromising nutritional integrity. Incorporating a diverse array of calcium sources, including dairy and non-dairy options, diversifies nutrient intake and accommodates dietary preferences and restrictions. Likewise, integrating a spectrum of vitamin D-rich foods such as fatty fish, fortified dairy alternatives, and eggs bolsters calcium absorption and fosters bone strength. Moreover, stocking up on vitamin K sources like kale, spinach, broccoli, and fermented foods augments bone mineralization and fracture prevention efforts. By proactively replenishing kitchen supplies with bone-building foods, individuals can cultivate an environment conducive to optimal bone health and longevity, laying the groundwork for comprehensive osteoporosis management through nutrition.

CHAPTER 10
LIFESTYLE TIPS FOR STRONGER BONES

Maintaining strong and healthy bones is crucial for overall well-being and quality of life, especially as one ages. Several lifestyle factors play significant roles in bone health, and adopting appropriate habits can help prevent conditions like osteoporosis.

A balanced diet rich in essential nutrients, regular exercise, exposure to sunlight for adequate vitamin D synthesis, stress management techniques, and avoiding habits detrimental to bone health are key components of a bone-friendly lifestyle.

Exercise and Physical Activity Recommendations

Physical activity is fundamental for bone health as it stimulates bone formation and strengthens existing bone tissue. Weight-bearing exercises, such as walking, jogging, dancing, and strength training, are particularly beneficial for bones.

These activities help load the bones, stimulating them to become stronger and denser over time. Resistance exercises, such as lifting weights or using resistance bands, also help improve bone density by putting stress on the bones, triggering them to adapt and become stronger. Incorporating a variety of exercises into one's routine, including both weight-bearing and resistance exercises, is essential for maximizing bone health.

Sunlight Exposure For Vitamin D Synthesis

Vitamin D is crucial for bone health as it helps the body absorb calcium, a mineral essential for bone strength. Sunlight exposure is the primary source of vitamin D synthesis in the body.

When the skin is exposed to sunlight, it produces vitamin D through a series of chemical reactions. However, factors such as geographical location, season, time of day, skin pigmentation, and the use of sunscreen can affect the body's ability to produce vitamin D from sunlight. Therefore, spending time outdoors regularly, especially during peak sunlight hours and without sunscreen for short periods, can help maintain adequate vitamin D levels. In regions with limited sunlight or during the winter months, supplementation may be necessary to ensure optimal vitamin D levels.

Stress Management And Bone Health

Chronic stress can have detrimental effects on bone health by increasing the body's production of cortisol, a hormone that can lead to bone loss over time. Moreover, stress often contributes to unhealthy coping behaviors such as poor dietary choices, sedentary lifestyle habits, and inadequate sleep, all of which can further compromise bone health.

Therefore, implementing stress management techniques is essential for maintaining strong and healthy bones. Practices such as mindfulness meditation, deep breathing exercises, yoga, and progressive muscle relaxation can help reduce stress levels and promote overall well-being. Additionally, prioritizing self-care activities, maintaining a healthy work-life balance, and seeking support from friends, family, or mental health professionals can also contribute to better stress management and improved bone health.

Certain lifestyle habits can negatively impact bone health and increase the risk of osteoporosis and fractures. These include smoking, excessive alcohol consumption, and consuming a diet high in sodium and processed foods while low in calcium and vitamin D. Smoking has been linked to decreased bone density and increased fracture risk due to its detrimental effects on bone-forming cells and hormone levels. Similarly, excessive alcohol intake can interfere with calcium absorption and bone remodeling processes, leading to weaker bones over time. Additionally, a diet high in sodium can increase calcium excretion through urine, while inadequate intake of calcium and vitamin D can impair bone formation and maintenance. Therefore, avoiding these bone-detrimental habits and adopting a balanced diet rich in calcium, vitamin D, and other essential nutrients, along with moderate alcohol consumption and abstaining from smoking, are crucial for preserving bone health and reducing the risk of osteoporosis.

CONCLUSION

the (Osteoporosis Diet Cookbook) offers a comprehensive guide to managing osteoporosis through nutrition, recipes, meal plans, and lifestyle strategies for optimal bone health. By incorporating the principles outlined in the cookbook, individuals can take proactive steps toward preventing osteoporosis and maintaining strong and healthy bones throughout their lives. Lifestyle factors such as regular exercise, adequate sunlight exposure for vitamin D synthesis, stress management techniques, and avoiding bone-detrimental habits play crucial roles in supporting bone health. Through education, awareness, and the implementation of evidence-based practices, individuals can empower themselves to prioritize bone health and enhance their overall quality of life.